Sex Change — Male to Female

*An Essential Guide
to Understanding
the Process of Gender
Reassignment Surgery
and Getting to Know
the New You*

by Eleanor Nye

Table of Contents

Introduction

Sex change surgery is a life-changing decision that has to be thoroughly considered and thought through. However, if you've reached the point of hating yourself for being male, or where being male is negatively affecting your mental and emotional health, then perhaps a male to female (MTF) sex change is the right step for you in order to feel like a more authentic version of yourself.

Before you proceed, there are some vital facts that you should know. The process is not as simple and straightforward as you might think. There are rules implemented by the World Professional Association for Transgender Health (WPATH) before any surgery can be performed. It's crucial that you learn about all of this so that you can come to an informed decision. Also, you should fully consider the permanent and irreversible changes that the gender reassignment surgery can have on your total persona.

This book is designed to provide you with valuable information that will help you better understand the process and be prepared for what's in store. It also includes a summary of the steps that you can follow in your gender reassignment process, including estimates for the cost of the surgery, along with other additional tips and pointers that will help guide you towards a successful transformation into a woman — the real you!

Chapter 1: Understanding the Process of Sex Change Surgery

Gender reassignment surgery or sex change surgery is a complex process that you have to fully understand. If you have decided to change your gender from male to female, you have to know all the procedures that are involved.

What is sex change surgery?

Sex change surgery is an invasive process where a surgeon operates on a person to change his or her gender. It involves a series of surgeries to change the secondary sexual characteristics of a person to that of the gender that he/she aspires to be. In your case, that will be from male to female (MTF).

What are the surgical procedures commonly performed for MTF surgeries?

The primary goal is to transform you from your current male gender into female. There are several female physical traits that you don't have as a male, and it would take a series of operations to construct these female parts in your body. You may opt to undergo all of these surgeries or just select some; it's up to you.

1. **Penectomy**—This is the surgical division of the penis into 3 pieces to give way for the construction of the vagina (vaginoplasty), specifically the vaginal canal and the clitoris. Getting rid of the penis will eliminate the ultimate symbol of masculinity and male gender from your body.

2. **Vaginoplasty**—As a trans female, having a vagina can boost your self- confidence. The vagina is one the major female sexual organs. Doing away with your penis and having a vagina will make you feel more feminine. This is done by using the tissue from the penis and

the scrotum in constructing the vagina and the labia. Tampon dilators will aid in making your newly-constructed vagina wider and deeper. As you engage in sexual intercourse with your new vagina, it will stretch and make the sensations more genuine.

3. **Vulvoplasty**—The vagina is incomplete without the vulva (lips) composed of the labia majora (outer lips) and the labia minora (inner lips). Without the vulva, your vagina will appear as an unpleasant looking opening. If you decide to undergo vaginoplasty, then you should also have vulvoplasty. In this operation, the tissues from the penectomy and the scrotum are used to construct the vulva.

4. **Breast implantation**—Aside from the vagina, the breasts are secondary sexual characteristics that you should possess as a transsexual. Those soft, and warm body parts will also enhance your figure as a female. Most of the growth of your breast will be due to your cross sex-hormone therapy or HRT, and you may prefer to stick to hormone therapy alone. But for bigger breasts, surgeons can perform breast augmentation or implants after

2 years of hormone therapy. So this is one major surgery you may want to choose. In this procedure, the surgeon will implant a synthetic material or silicon to augment your new breasts.

5. **Clitoroplasty**—If you want to increase your sexual sensations, you can choose to undergo clitoroplasty, the construction of your clitoris. Though the sensual pleasure is not assured to be a hundred percent, this surgery may succeed in allowing you to experience the same sensations that one of the centers of the female erotic zones provide. It's constructed on the previous nerve endings of the penis to simulate the sexual pleasures produced by penile stimulation. You may not know it, but sex experts have labeled the clitoris the female penis because of its similar erotic response to touch.

6. **Orchidectomy**—This involves the surgical removal of the testes. A uterus may be created in its place, depending on the surgeon's evaluation. This procedure is still being perfected, but you can inquire from your own surgeon about it.

7. **Facial reconstruction**—This also deals with aesthetic surgery, in which your male facial features are made more feminine. This will depend on your preferences, so choose wisely, which facial features you want to improve on. People will still consider your "face value" when assessing you. A beautiful feminine face can help a lot in your successful transformation from male to female.

These are the major MTF surgeries that you can choose from when deciding on your sex change surgery. Other minor procedures are body hair removal, waistline reduction and hair enhancement. The surgeries above can only be performed after you have prepared yourself properly and have fulfilled the criteria required. These will be discussed in the following chapter.

Chapter 2: Gender Reassignment Surgery Criteria

The WPATH and the Endocrine Society have set certain requirements to qualify individuals for sex reassignment surgery.

Here's a list of the requirements:

1. **The individual is certified to be suffering from persistent Gender Dysphoria**

   You must be certified as a persistent Gender Dysphoric person, by a competent health specialist licensed to provide certifications. Take note that being a homosexual is different from having Gender Dysphoria. In homosexuality, there's an acceptance of one's gender, while in Gender Dysphoria, there's a rejection of one's gender.

Gender Dysphoria is characterized by various symptoms, such as disgust and embarrassment over one's own birth gender, a persistent desire to be the opposite sex, and engagement in activities of the opposite gender. The person grows increasingly embarrassed and depressed as he/she becomes identified with his birth gender. The desire usually lasts 6 months or more, and becomes stronger as the individual becomes older. It's as if your female gender is trapped inside your male body.

NOTE: For more information about Gender Dysphoria:
www.amazon.com/dp/B0128EAGYU/ke ywords=gender+dysphoria

2. The person must be 18 years or older

This means that you must be an adult and have the authority to decide on your own. In special cases that concern children, the guardian or parent has to decide. Generally, children are not recommended to undergo sex change surgeries unless the condition is life-threatening. As an adult, you're expected to have decided wisely, and that there will be no regrets later on.

3. The person has no existing diseases, such as:

*   **Cardiac diseases**

    People with cardiac conditions can encounter complications when undergoing the series of MTF gender reassignment surgeries. It's not a one-time process, so it can be tedious, stressful and physically demanding, which can exacerbate the condition of persons with cardiac illnesses, such as a rheumatic heart, increased risk of myocardial infarction (heart attack) and cerebrovascular accidents (stroke).

*   **Diabetes**

    Diabetes mellitus (DM) is a condition caused by the insufficiency of insulin in the body, and is characterized by hyperglycemia (increased concentration of glucose or sugar in the blood), polyuria (increased urination), polydipsia (excessive thirst) and polyphagia (extreme hunger). Persons with diabetes may encounter complications, such as poor wound healing after a surgery that can cause infections of the wound, and necrosis of the surrounding tissues. DM is one of the most common causes for amputations of the legs due to tissue necrosis. For sure, you will want to ensure that your newly-implanted breasts are not excised because the surgical wounds won't heal.

- **Hepatitis**

Hepatitis is a blood borne disease caused by the different types of hepatitis virus, A, B, C, D and E. It's infectious, so surgeons have to take special precautions when performing any type of surgery. Typically, the doctor will treat you first for your hepatitis before any sex change surgery is performed. In some cases, your doctor may not recommend surgery at all. This will depend upon the type and severity of your hepatitis infection.

- **Human Immunodeficiency Virus (HIV) infection or Acute Immunodeficiency Syndrome (AIDS)**

This is also a blood borne infectious disease, which is caused by the impairment of a person's immune system by HIV. When a person's body defenses are down, he can contract any illness that he's exposed to. The condition has no cure but the symptoms can be treated. The doctor will recommend treatment of your HIV complications and will discourage you from entertaining the idea of a sex change.

- **Mental illness**

Becoming a trans female doesn't only involve MTF sex change surgeries but also the complete conversion of your mind-set from male to female. If you have a mental illness, this process will be difficult for you. You have to possess a normal functioning brain to be able to use your mental powers effectively. Your mind has a major function in your successful transformation from male to female because the brain is the center of your Central Nervous System (CNS) and is responsible in "commanding" how your body should react and behave.

- **Breast cancer**

Yes, men can also have breast cancer. If you have breast cancer, it's a given that gender reassignment surgery is not recommended. Depending on the stage of the cancer, constructing new breasts on top of the affected area will only worsen the spread of the cancer cells. Surgical procedures may also worsen your disease.

4. **The person is apparently healthy**

In a nutshell, you must be apparently healthy with no serious pathological diseases. This will help ensure that the sex change surgery will have no complications.

5. One year of continuous hormone therapy

Before the surgery, you must have taken feminizing hormones for a year. The Hormone Replacement Therapy (HRT) involves estrogen and progesterone. Some examples of hormones used for HRT are conjugated estrogen and Ethinyloestradiol or Ethinyl Estradiol.

Conjugated estrogen of 7.5 to 10 milligrams per deciliter (mg/dL) is usually administered. Another example is 100 µg (micrograms) of Ethinyloestradiol. This can also be given daily in two separate doses. The dosage can be increased to 150 µg daily depending on your response. These female hormones will aid in developing your secondary female sexual characteristics. The dosage can be reduced to 50 µg after 6 to 12 months of hormone therapy.

Cross hormone therapy may continue one week after the sex change surgery and can be discontinued or continued depending on the recommendations of your health specialist. Normally, hormones exert their effects gradually, but overdosing can also result in serious conditions, such as cancer and tumors. Hence, beware of these harmful side effects.

Side effects of hormonal therapy:

- **Infertility**—You can become sterile after becoming a transgender.

- **Formation of gall stones**—These stones can cause obstruction that may require surgery.

- **Sleep apnea**—You can experience sleep disturbances that will affect your health.

- **Venous thrombosis or blood clot formation**—There's an increased risk of blood clot formation that can block arteries and cause death. This is the reason why estrogen therapy must be stopped three to four weeks before the scheduled surgery.

- **Obesity**—Some people become obese because of hormonal replacement therapy. This is heightened by genetic and environmental factors.

- **Acne**—Increased concentrations of sexual hormones can cause acne, especially in young adults.

6. The person has actively lived as a trans female for one year

Real life experience is an essential requirement that you have to undergo before the sex reassignment surgery. You should live and engage in the daily activities of females for at least one year. This is the crucial trial period to determine that you're definitely comfortable living as a female transsexual.

7. The person has to undergo psychotherapy for at least a year

You have to visit your psychotherapist for a year to condition your mind and body to your impending MTF transformation. The psychotherapist will assist you in resolving issues about your gender identity problem and will evaluate whether you are, indeed, Gender Dysphoric. The diagnosis can be done together with a competent team of specialists that may include a psychiatrist, psychologist, medical doctor and a sex therapist.

8. Two certificates from the psychotherapist and the doctor (endocrinologist)

Sex change surgery requires these two certificates to confirm your Gender Dysphoric status and to ensure that you don't have hormonal disorders. Without these two certificates, you won't be able to undergo gender reassignment in a legitimate sex change center.

These are all the pre-requisites needed for you to qualify for a sex change surgery. Go over them and determine if you're able to meet all the requirements. If you do, then you can proceed to the next step.

Chapter 3: Post-Surgery Precautions to Observe

After the surgery, you have to observe certain precautions to prevent complications from occurring. Keep in mind, that it takes a series of surgical procedures before you can become a female. Just as there are requirements and precautions before the surgery, which are presented in Chapter 2, there are also precautions observed after the sex change surgery.

After-surgery precautions:

1. **Continuous psychotherapy and counseling**

    Your psychotherapy and counseling must continue until such time that you're fully adjusted to the new you. The psychotherapist will help in your transformation to your new gender and likewise, assist you in your psychological problems concerning your transgender conversion after the surgery.

2. Continuous hormone therapy

For MTF transsexuals, the estrogen therapy has to continue until the doctor recommends cessation of the therapy. In previous cases, there were instances where the growth of skin hair increased when the administration of feminizing hormones stopped. In the event that you have to prolong your intake of the hormone, remember to monitor your blood hormone levels to ensure that they're within normal limits appropriate for your trans-female status.

3. Performing activities that enhance your female gender

Having a successful sex change surgery is not enough to ensure that your transformation is complete. Don't just stop there—enjoy activities that enhance your acceptance of belonging to the female gender, like delicate hobbies (e.g. crochet), experimenting with hair accessories, pampering yourself with facials and manicures, or adding hair extensions with soft, gorgeous curls.

More ways to enhance your new female gender are presented in Chapter 6.

Chapter 4: How Much Does It Cost?

Now, that you're all set and qualified to undergo a sex change surgery, you may be interested in knowing how much it would cost. The cost varies significantly, from as low as $80.00 to as high as $150,000. Typically, male to female sex change surgeries are less expensive than the other way around. The price will depend on the number of surgeries you intend to undergo. Remember to include the expenses incurred for your psychotherapy and hormone therapy before and after the surgery as well.

Here's a rough estimate of the cost of a sex change procedure from MTF.

Psychotherapy for one year before the surgery— $100 per session per week

$100 (per session) x 4 weeks x 12 months = **$4,800**

**Total of pre-treatment psychotherapy =
$2,400/**year

After the surgery, the doctor may give the hormone for a lifetime or for a few months. He may also adjust the amount of hormones administered.

Let's say you're 45 years old now, and the doctor has decided that you must take the hormones for a lifetime. Assuming that your hormone therapy costs the same as your psychotherapy, if you live up to 65 years old, the computation of your hormone therapy expenses will be:

65 years - 45 years = 20 years x $2,400 (one year) = $48,000

Plus one year pre-treatment before surgery = $2,400

Grand total = $50,400.00

Surgical procedures:

$30,000 to $40,000

Total cost:

The total cost will be **$95, 200**. This includes the following:

- Pre-Psychotherapy = $2,400

- Post-Psychotherapy = $2,400

- Pre and post-hormonal treatment = $50,400

- Surgery = $40,000

You can opt for discounted packages offered by sex change centers, or you can also search for gender reassignment doctors through the TSSurgeryguide.com (http://www.tssurgeryguide.com/SRS-Surgeon-Ratings.html). This site provides a list of qualified doctors, who can perform the surgery in the US.

In Trinidad, Colorado, there are a number of sex change centers you can visit and explore. Visit each center and select the one that offers procedures that adhere to your preferences and needs.

If you're a student, there are also American universities who offer a myriad of services to students and parents who plan to become transsexuals. While some universities have limited transsexual programs, the University of Illinois Urbana has already included sex change surgery in its health insurance program. Some universities that offer this service are the Universities of Northwestern, Duke, Yale and Stanford.

In line with the WPATH goal, the University of Michigan Health System followed suit with its Comprehensive Gender Services Program (UMHS-

CGSP). This program allows parents and students to avail of its Sex Reassignment Surgeries (SRS).

If you live in the UK, you can visit the Transhealth center on their website http://www.transhealth.co.uk/. Alternatively, you can travel to Thailand or Iran, where the majority of sex change surgeries are performed and explore the reliability of those services.

Finding a sex change center in your area would, however, be more convenient and would reduce your costs (no traveling expenses).

Take note of the adage "Haste makes waste", so search judiciously and evaluate all the services before signing up with any of these sex change centers. Your primary consideration should always be your health.

Chapter 5: The Benefits of Gender Reassignment

For Gender Dysphoric persons, gender reassignment surgery is definitely beneficial. This is because it's the appropriate solution to their problems. If you're a Gender Dysphoric person, who has finally decided to become a trans female, here are the specific benefits you can enjoy.

1. **Elimination of depression and anxiety caused by discomfort with your gender**

    You will no longer feel depressed and anxious about your gender because you will now feel more at home in your own body. Gender Dysphoric persons even feel repulsed about their birth gender, and becoming a trans female will help solve this problem.

2. More self-confidence

Since you'll be more comfortable with your female traits, you'll be more self-confident about yourself. You'll love who you are, so you'll project this aura to other people.

3. Advancement in career

You'll also be able to advance in your career because of your newly-acquired self-confidence.

4. Improvement in personal relationships

Everything falls into place when you're happy, confident and comfortable with your gender and yourself. By being true to yourself, your relationships will improve. You're no longer hiding your true identity and people who love and like you, do so with their eyes open. The fear of discovery is no longer hovering above your head like a Damocles sword. You'll feel a sense of relief, be at peace and feel stress-free for the first time in a very long time.

5. Staying true to one's self

You will no longer live a lie, and you will be able to stay true to yourself. You'll be an authentic woman in your mind, body and soul.

These are the advantages that you can reap when you decide to undergo gender reassignment surgery.

If you have followed properly the pre and post-surgical pointers, the other foreseeable disadvantages will most probably include your experience of discrimination as a transsexual. You can overcome this by being self-confident about who you are and by knowing your rights. Another disadvantage is that not all insurance policies cover sex change surgeries. Refer to Chapter 4 for more information.

Chapter 6: 9 Steps in the Sex Change Process

Here is the summary of the steps that you need to take if you're going to undertake a sex change:

Step #1—Consult a psychotherapist and a doctor

This is the first step to determine whether you have Gender Dysphoria or not. The psychotherapist will base his diagnosis on your medical history and symptoms, while the doctor will rule out other underlying illnesses with the same symptoms using diagnostic tests. You should be diagnosed as a Gender Dysphoric person for the psychotherapist to issue a letter of recommendation for your gender reassignment surgery.

NOTE: For more information about Gender Dysphoria: www.amazon.com/dp/B0128EAGYU/keywords =gender+dysphoria

Step #2—Make the final decision

Once you've obtained the recommendation from the health specialists, you must assess yourself if you're committed to the sex change surgery. If you have Gender Dysphoria, a sex change surgery is the best resolution to your problem because you'll never be able to accept your birth gender. However, you have to commit yourself completely to the process.

Step #3—Undertake continuous psychotherapy for 1 year

As discussed in Chapters 2 and 3, this is one of the requirements before a person undergoes surgery. This process will ensure that you're mentally and psychologically prepared.

Step #4—Consult an endocrinologist

This step is done to determine if your hormone therapy is appropriate or not. The blood concentration of the female hormones, estrogen and progesterone are measured, together with your testosterone and androgens. The endocrinologist will recommend the appropriate hormone therapy for you.

Step #5—Undergo hormone replacement therapy (HRT) for 1 year

You will take feminizing hormones for 1 year to develop your female secondary sexual characteristics. These are: broadening of hips, development of breasts, reduction of skin hair, reduction of a muscular built, and in some instances, a change to a higher-pitched voice. Additional facts about HRT are presented in the topics where they are specifically referred to (Chapters 2 and 3).

Step #6—Exposure to real life experience as a transgender for 1 year

While you're undergoing psychotherapy and HRT, you can simultaneously undergo the real life experience of living as a female transgender. You should experience all the activities that your future gender undergoes on a daily basis.

Step #7—Undergo the sex change surgeries

You're now prepared to proceed with your sex change surgeries. Understand that these operations will occur through a period of time. It will take years for you to fully undergo all the needed surgical interventions for your transformation.

Step #8—Continue with psychotherapy and HRT until necessary

After the surgery, you still have to continue with your psychotherapy and hormone therapy as recommended by your team of health specialists.

Step #9—Live your life as a woman

After all the surgical procedures are completed, you can now start living your life as a woman.

These are the major steps that you can do to become a trans woman. Be guided accordingly.

Chapter 7: Getting to Know the New You

You've successfully transformed into the new you. Now you're ready to go out there and conquer the world. One of the most important things to remember is that your transformation must include all aspects of your personality: physical, mental and psychological aspects. The brain is a powerful tool that you can effectively use to get to know the new you. Remember to use it wisely. Here are guides you can use in this process.

1. Accept the new you fully

You may have always wished that you could become a female, and now that your dream has come true, you may still have doubts. You must psyche yourself that you have now attained your dream and everything is real. Hence, you have to accept this new identity. Every morning, look at the mirror and mentally or say "This is the new me. I'm happy about it and I accept this new me" out loud.

2. Love the new you

No one can love the new you if you don't love her yourself. The love you show yourself will rebound to other people around you and they'll want to love the new you, as well.

3. Apply for a new name

Getting to know the new "you' means assigning a new feminine name. Your psychotherapists and the team of health specialists that have done your surgery can issue certificates attesting to the fact that you're a transsexual. These certificates can act as evidence for you to obtain a court order change or a Gender Recognition Certificate (GRC). The court order will allow you to legally change your name and your gender. You have to refer to the federal laws existing in your own country or state for the specifics. While you're applying for a new name, you can also apply for a new driver's license and passport.

4. Enlist the support of family and friends

Your family members and close friends are good support systems. Explain to them why you had to undergo sex change and express your need for their love, understanding and support. Request that your doctor explain to them the need for your surgery. Your loved ones will surely understand. A tap on the back, an encouraging word or two from them will go a long way in helping you welcome the new you.

5. Join support groups

Members who have undergone the same procedures as you have can help you with your new gender identity. You can learn from their experiences and you can also share some tips with them. They will help you get to know the new you.

6. Be courageous to socialize

You need to socialize and come out of your shell. People can only hurt you if you allow them to. Let them know that you're not ashamed to be a transsexual and that you're confident with who you are, because you like who you are.

These are the techniques in getting to know the new you. You already know who you are as a person, and the new you has the same character as the old you, only possessing the opposite gender—the more feminine version of you.

Chapter 8: Traits to Develop as a Female

You now belong to the female gender, and you don't have to be a rocket scientist to know the traits that you should develop as a female. It's pretty obvious, right? BUT many trans females may still be groping in the dark about what's expected from them. A lot of men say that "women are difficult to understand"; hence, this chapter will help you learn more about the female gender.

1. Feminine voice

There are voice therapy or voice training lessons offered for MTF transsexuals. These voice feminization trainings will aid you in doing away with your previous masculine vocals. Vocal surgery may or may not change your voice, so voice therapy is recommended instead because it's safer and non-invasive. You can also enlist the help of a speech therapist, or a speech pathologist to feminize your voice.

2. "Queenly" attributes

While women fight for equality, the majority of women still want to be with men, who would open doors for them and offer them a seat on a crowded bus. They want men to be their knights in shining armor and treat them as queens. So, as a woman, choose a gentleman to be with. Act as a queen, maintaining your poise and elegance. People will respect you if you observe good manners and appropriate conduct. On the other hand, don't act like a spoiled brat or a pompous diva because people will avoid you. Think of yourself as a woman of good breeding and you'll act accordingly.

3. Vanity (consciousness about facial appearance)

The majority of females are more conscious of their faces than men. As the cliché goes: "Woman, thy name is vanity." You should learn how to apply makeup to enhance your feminine features. You can go to a beauty salon to ask for advice in applying your makeup until you become more adept at it yourself. You can apply simple makeup, such as a dash of lipstick or a bit of blush every time you go out. This is a skill that you can easily acquire as a woman. Also, your beautician can add eyelash extensions and permanent feminine eyebrows to make your eyes appear more soulful and feminine. Don't worry, with practice you can apply makeup just as easily as you can wink your eyes. You may even prefer no makeup, which is just as valid an option.

4. Emotional strength

It's believed that women are emotionally stronger than men, while men are physically dominant. Of course, there will always be exceptions to this, but, although women cry more than men, they're considered emotionally stronger.

5. Smoother skin

Women have naturally smoother skin. Your anti-androgenic hormones or female hormones will aid in the prevention of skin and facial hair growth. Nevertheless, having constant hair removal and skin treatment at a beauty salon can significantly smoothen your skin and prevent hair growth in unwanted areas. An armpit hair laser treatment can result in hairless and smooth armpits.

These are some of the feminine traits that you may want to enhance. Remember that every person has both female and male characteristics, and it's up to you to enhance the feminine side because that's who you want to be.

Chapter 9: Coping with Transsexuality

Undergoing that long awaited surgery and finally becoming a female is a multifarious process. The pre and post-surgical procedures are also varied, so you need all the information you can glean to ensure that your transformation is successful. The following are suggestions that can be useful in your endeavor.

1. **Have a positive frame of mind.** You're halfway to success if you're an optimist. This is due to the fact that people who are positive can overcome problems more easily. They know how to persevere and keep going despite failures.

2. **You may encounter discrimination as a transsexual.** There have been some reports of discrimination when a person was revealed to be transsexual. Know your rights. Each state or country has laws regarding the non-discrimination of transsexuals.

3. **Trans females have a legitimate gender.** If you're told otherwise, don't be bothered. You're a female and no one can take that away from you.

4. **If you're serious about a relationship, be honest.** Truth will always prevail, so reveal your transsexual experience with your beloved. If he truly loves you, nothing else will matter.

5. **Transsexuals are included under transgenders.** Transsexuals are those who have undergone sex gender reassignment, while transgenders encompass transsexuals, and all other types of gender deviation, who may not want to undergo sex change surgeries.

6. **Internationally, you can refer to the WPATH for other information.** This organization has members all over the world that can assist you become a legitimate transsexual.

7. **Cross Hormone Therapy or HRT may not be enough to develop breasts**. In this case, you need breast augmentation to complete the procedure. The majority of trans women prefer to undergo breast augmentation or implantation.

8. **Even if you have Gender Dysphoria, you may opt not to undertake sex change surgery.** It's still a voluntary process. You have the final say about the surgery you want done on YOUR body.

9. **Gender reassignment is a gradual process.** It takes years of complex therapy and surgical methods for your complete transformation from male to female. So, be mentally, physically and financially prepared.

10. **In male to female sex changes, your prostate is usually retained.** Scientists are still in the process of perfecting the method to remove the prostate gland and replacing it with the ovaries.

11. **Sexual orientation is different from Gender Dysphoria.** Sexual orientation involves your sexual preferences, while Gender Dysphoria involves what gender you truly want to be.

NOTE: For more information about Gender Dysphoria:
www.amazon.com/dp/B0128EAGYU/ke ywords=gender+dysphoria

12. **Male to female (MTF) sex reassignment surgery is cheaper than female to male (FTM).** But, be ready for contingencies. It pays to have extra cash in the bank, in case an emergency happens.

These are useful pointers you can use in the course of your transformation. Add this list to your previous knowledge and get the most out of the information.

Conclusion

Sex change surgery from male to female is a complex process. It will take years for the transformation to be complete. But, the sure thing is that you can finally become a woman, if you persist in your efforts and follow the information presented in this book.

Once you've decided to undergo your gender reassignment surgery, you have to stand by your decision through thick and thin. There should be no going back and no reluctance to undergo all the required procedures.

After your series of surgeries, when you have already become a woman, be proud of yourself and relish your gender because you have released yourself from the clutches of your birth gender.

Have fun and enjoy your life as a new woman!

Finally, I'd like to thank you for purchasing this book! If you found it helpful, I'd greatly appreciate it if you'd take a moment to leave a review on Amazon. Thank you!

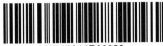

27516244R00039

Printed in Great Britain
by Amazon